A Guide to Medicinal Wild Fruits & Berries

Written and Illustrated by
Julie Gomez

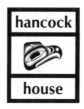

hancock
house

ISBN 0-88839-445-4
Copyright © 1999 Julie Gomez

Cataloging in Publication Data
Gomez, Julie, 1964–
  A guide to medicinal wild fruits & berries

  ISBN 0-88839-445-4

  1. Fruit--Identification. 2. Fruit--Therapeutic use.
  3. Berries--Identification. 4. Berries--Therapeutic use.
  5. Medicinal plants. I. Title.
  QK99.A1G65 1999   581.4'64   C98-911040-0

Editor: Nancy Miller
Production: Ingrid Luters

Published simultaneously in Canada and the United States by

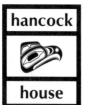

HANCOCK HOUSE PUBLISHERS LTD.
19313 Zero Avenue, Surrey, B.C. V4P 1M7
(604) 538-1114 Fax (604) 538-2262

HANCOCK HOUSE PUBLISHERS
1431 Harrison Avenue, Blaine, WA 98230
(604) 538-1114 Fax (604) 538-2262
Web Site: www.hancockhouse.com *email:* sales@hancockhouse.com

Contents

Botanical Glossary

Axil: The V-shaped angle between the stalk and the stem where they join.

Berry: Deriving from a plant's ripened ovary or ovaries, contains soft or hard seeds loosely embedded within its pulp, and has no stone.

Bloom: A white powdery film coating berries and leaves.

Bract: Small modified leaves near the flower.

Calyx: Fused or open sepals that support the flower.

Compound: A division of leaves that form a group of three or more.

Deciduous: Trees and shrubs that lose their leaves seasonally.

Fruit: Deriving from a plant's ripened ovary, ovaries or receptacles, contains a stone that encloses one or more seeds, and have seeds embedded within a fleshy core.

Herb: A succulent, nonwoody, seed-bearing plant that dies back yearly.

Lobe: The division of a leaf.

Margin: Leaf edges.

Midrib: The vein through the center of a leaf.

Naturalized: A non-native (introduced) plant species that is able to grow and spread, and behaves like a native species without human interference.

Nurse log: A downed tree that supports a foundation for new plant forms to take root.

Shrub: An evergreen or deciduous woody plant that has numerous trunks.

Stamen: The organ of a flower in which the pollen is held.

Tree: An evergreen or deciduous woody plant that generally produces a single trunk, although multiple trunks are common.

Medicinal Glossary

Antiseptic: An agent that purifies and cleanses.

Ointment: A semisolid mixture containing plant material(s) to be applied externally to portions of the body.
METHOD: One part powdered plant material(s) mixed with four parts petroleum jelly. Heat mixture and apply to skin.

Poultice: An external application of plant material that is applied to a portion of the body.
METHOD: Made from dried, powdered or fresh plant material(s) combined with hot water. If desired, a paste can be made by mixing oatmeal or flour with the plant material(s). The warmed herbal paste (called a plaster) is then placed between the folds of a warmed cheesecloth and applied to the inflamed or sore area of the skin. Change the cheesecloth when it cools and repeat as necessary.

Powder: Dried, crushed, plant material to be taken internally.

METHOD: Mix a coarse powder with eight-ounce glass of water or milk or add to soup. Usual dosage is one small pinch.

Tea: Dried or fresh plant material(s) steeped in hot water to be taken internally.

METHOD: Use one teaspoon of dried material(s) or two tablespoons of fresh plant material(s) for every six ounces of hot water. Steep in hot water for five to ten minutes and strain. If stronger tea is desired, add more plant material(s). Sweeten with honey. It is best to boil water in a non-metal pot and drink tea from glass or ceramic since aluminum and other metals can leach into the water.

Tincture: The soaking of plant material in alcohol and water to be taken as internal medicine.

METHOD: Used by the drop, and typically consists of one part alcohol (100 proof vodka is most commonly used) and one part water. Never use rubbing alcohol; it can be fatal if ingested. General use includes one to four ounces of fresh or dried plant material chopped and placed in a large amber jar and then covered with the liquid solution. Make sure plant material is completely covered then seal and label jar with the date and the name of its contents. Store out of direct sunlight and shake solution daily for two to six weeks. Solution may evaporate some, especially if using dried material. Add more alcohol as

necessary. At the end of two to six weeks, strain off plant material and store liquid in small amber bottles. Usual dosage is one drop to one tablespoon added to an eight-ounce glass of water or milk three times a day. (Hot water dissolves the tincture's alcohol but does not effect its potency.)

Tonic: A slow-acting stimulant that improves general health.

METHOD: Made using the same method as an herbal tea, but then stored in amber bottles for future use. Mild tonics can be taken on a daily basis. Store out of direct sunlight since this will destroy the herb's potency.

Wash: An external, liquid application containing plant material that is applied to a portion of the body.

METHOD: Use fresh plant amterials soaked in clean water; then remove them. The liquid is used as an eyewash or for treating earaches or itching and sunburn.

Warning! Some plants can cause burning or irritation when used as a poultice or ointment. Powders are generally very potent and should not be used over a long period of time (i.e., six months). Never use any plant material that hasn't been positively identified, because toxic poisoning can result. Consult a physician before using any plant as a medicine, tea, poultice or ointment.

For Brandon

Acknowledgments

I would like to thank the following for their generosity and help. Pacific Northwest Gardener for answering my questions concerning fruit and berry identification. The friendly staff of the Portland Nursery who answered my questions and who provided me with the native plant specimens I was looking for. Paul Slichter of the Gresham High School botany class who generously provided information on plant identification. My parents Bill and Patsy who have joined me on countless drives into the countryside, often stopping in an instant at my request, so that I could retrieve plant samples. Finally, I would like to thank my husband Christopher who accompanies me on many forest paths sampling, often hesitantly, nature's bountiful harvest.

Introduction

For many, berry picking is a wonderful, seasonal treat that gets a person outdoors into wild places in search of their favorite berry. For others, it summons the horror stories told of wild berries, sadly preventing one the experience of sampling beyond the blackberry thickets that line many a roadside.

Fruits and berries occur on trees, shrubs, vines and herbs. They begin to appear in midspring flaunting their colorful shapes against rich shades of forest green. By early summer their numbers increase, revealing more shades of yellows, reds, blues and purples among fertile woods and mountain meadows. It isn't until late fall that their numbers begin to dwindle. Some will persist throughout the winter, but usually in such low numbers that they are of little value to the berry picker.

It is common knowledge that fruits and berries are a savory treat. Even as I write, I sip on warmed cranberry tea sweetened with raspberry honey—delicious! Wild fruits and berries are considerably different from store-bought versions. Most have unique flavors that may or may not be appealing to the taste buds. Some are dry, extremely bitter and very seedy, and some will require seed removal and a sweetener to make them more enjoyable. Others may be sweet, juicy and pleasantly tart—needing nothing more than a little cream poured over top of them. As food, they often make wonderful substitutes or additions to a favorite recipe. Some common uses include jams, jellies, pies, puddings, raisins, salads, soups, stews, lemonade, lemon juice, flour, coffee and tea.

Fruits and berries are not only good to eat, but they also contain medicinal values that are both healthful and healing. Vitamin rich, they contain substantial amounts of vitamins A, B2 (riboflavin) and C, as well as fiber, iron, potassium, magnesium, beta carotene, malic and citric acids, and essential oils that the body requires to stay healthy. For example, if suffering from constipation, the fresh fruits of the wood strawberry (*Fragaria vesca*) acts as a mild laxative if eaten in quantity, lessen the quantity and the fruit relieves diarrhea. It also promotes urine flow, and its juices have a remarkable cooling effect. Another species, the red huckleberry (*Vaccinium parvifolium*) has wonderful tasting berries that when dried and prepared as tea can relieve diarrhea. Its juice acts as an appetite stimulant.

Also having medicinal value, as well as being vitamin rich, are the plants that produce the fruit. Depending on the species, the root, bark, leaves, flowers and oils all produce various amounts of vitamins A, B complex, C, E and K as well as generate calcium, iron, copper and magnesium. As food, some common uses include potherbs, fritters, pickles, sugar, flour, lemonade, coffee and tea. As for medicinal value, these are many and varied. For example, the leaves of false Soloman's seal (*Smilacina racemosa*) can be used as an external wash to relieve itching. The flowers of the flowering dogwood (*Cornus florida*) can be used fresh or dried for making tea to relieve diarrhea, indigestion, fever and symptoms of pneumonia.

Before we venture outdoors to partake from nature's pharmacy, I must first mention some rules of safety. **Before using any plant material for medicinal purposes, always consult a licensed practitioner**. Self diagnosis should never be attempted. This book is not a prescriptor and should not be used as such. Avoid collecting roadside vegetation where traffic is heavy or where chemical sprays have been used, as toxic poisoning can result. Never assume a fruit or berry is safe to eat because birds or other animals were seen feeding on them; such an assumption could be your last. Poisonous species can sometimes resemble harmless look-alikes, especially when they are without their fruits or berries. They may also contain both edible and poisonous parts so know what you are collecting. Remember, if there is the slightest doubt—leave it!

A word about collecting. For conservation purposes most state and provincial parks strictly prohibit berry picking in quantity; however, sampling one here and there is usually all right. The removal of park vegetation is strictly prohibited and, if ignored, heavy fines can result. A good way to legally harvest plant material from the wild is to salvage them (with permission of course) from a site where the land is to be bulldozed for future development. Many of the plant specimens collected for this book were salvaged from such lands. Never trespass onto private property without getting permission first. When collecting, always cut plant materials never tear them; if digging is required, use a shovel and fill in the hole afterwards. Avoid trampling an area excessively to have as little an impact on the landscape as possible so that others may also enjoy the wild benefits.

What about tools? For picking soft fruits and berries I recommend using a flat basket to keep them from getting crushed, otherwise a bucket with a handle will do nicely. Small garden clippers are essential for collecting vegetation, make sure that they are sharp so clean cuttings will result. Wear gloves if handling thorny vegetation to avoid cuts and scratches and contact with plant juices that can sometimes irritate the skin. Transport vegetation in burlap sacks or paper bags. Avoid plastic since it tends to trap moisture, causing easy spoilage.

Whatever the ailment, nature can provide the remedy. Just remember, whether collecting for food or for medicine a little common sense and careful selection will make your experience of wild food foraging fun, but most importantly, it will make it safe. See you beyond the blackberry thickets!

Black Hawthorn *Crataegus douglasii*

Flowers: white; bloom May–June.
Fruit: reddish black; September–November.
Life cycle: deciduous tree or shrub.
Size: ten to sixteen feet tall.

This familiar tree or shrub is known for its wicked, one-inch, needlelike thorns and dense foliage. Its bark is gray and generally smooth in young plants, while older plants are rough and furrowed. Leaves alternate and measure one to two inches long. They are dark green above and pale green below with prominent veins. They are shallow lobed with toothed margins and are broadly ovate with a narrow leaf base. Their texture is thick and leathery. Flowers are small, white, five-petalled and measure one-quarter inch to one-half inch long. Flavor quality is poor to fair as they are mildly sweet, somewhat tart and slightly bland. Seeds are hard nutlets that number two to five.

Habitat: forest edges, thickets, stream banks, roadsides.

Medicinal parts: flowers, berries.

Harvest: late spring–early summer, flowers; fall, berries.

Medicinal uses: fresh flower or berry tea tincture for diarrhea, skin disorders, sore throats, high or low blood pressure, heart murmur, artery spasms, to promote urine flow.

Warning! Watch out when gathering the flowers and berries of this plant. Its thorns are long and extremely sharp, and serious wounds can result.

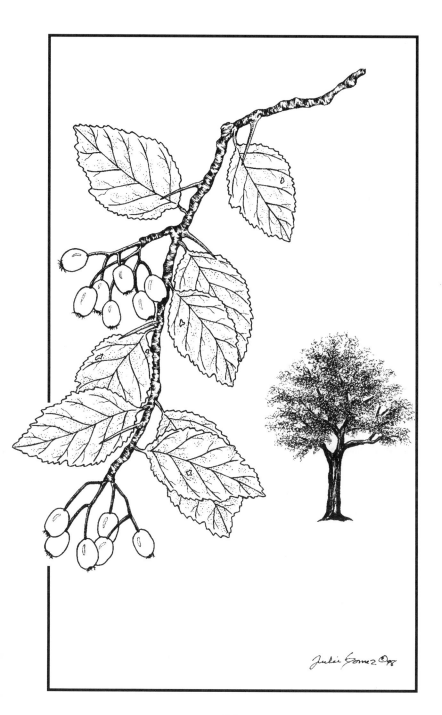

Julie Gomez ©98

Pacific Crabapple *Malus fusca*

Flowers: white to pink; bloom May–June.
Fruit: green to yellow to red; August–September.
Life cycle: deciduous tree.
Size: to thirty feet tall.

Bark is dark brown and usually smooth in young trees; older trees are rough and scaly. Leaves alternate and measure two to three and one-half inches long. They are dark green above, grayish green below (usually hairy) and have a distinct, hairy midrib. Broadly ovate, they have pointed tips, a heart-shaped base and irregular, shallow-toothed margins. Long-stemmed, leaves are close together on rough, thorny twigs that often reveal numerous leaf scars. Twigs are thin with a slight velvety texture. Flowers are large, white- to pink-colored and measure one inch wide. They are five-petaled, very fragrant and appear in flat-topped, showy clusters. Fruit color ranges from green to yellow to deep red. They are oblong-shaped and measure one-half to three-quarters inch long. Their flavor is tart. Seeds are hard and located in the center of the core.

Habitat: coastal estuaries, swamps, bogs, moist woods, clearings, fields, thickets, lake edges, roadsides.

Medicinal parts: bark, leaves, buds, flowers, fruit.

Harvest: spring, bark, leaves, buds, flowers; late summer–fall, fruit.

Medicinal uses: bark tea or tincture for fever, nausea, diarrhea, internal parasites, bladder, kidney, spleen and colon disorders, inducing sleep; dried leaf, bud or flower tea for colds, sore throats, to promote urine flow; fresh, dried or cooked fruit for constipation, inducing sleep, cleansing liver, colon, spleen, kidneys and gall bladder; fruit pulp poultice for minor cuts and inflammation.

Warning! Bark, leaves and seeds contain various amounts of cyanide that can cause poisoning; use is not recommended. Sources indicate a person died after eating a cupful of seeds. Cooking is recommended as fruit can be hard to digest.

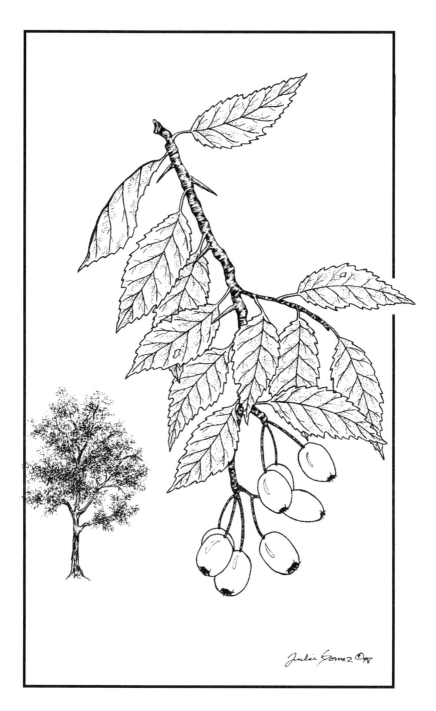

Julie Gomez ©98

European Mountain Ash   *Sorbus aucuparia*

Flowers: creamy white; bloom May–June
Fruit: yellow-orange to red; August–November.
Life cycle: deciduous tree or shrub.
Size: twenty to fifty feet tall.

Often planted as an ornamental, this fast-growing, short-lived tree (shrub) has naturalized successfully. Its bark is silver-gray to reddish brown and generally smooth in young trees, becoming rough and scaly with age. Leaves are compound and alternate. Leaflets are lance-shaped, number from nine to fifteen (per compound) and measure two inches. They are dark green above, white and hairy below. They have pointed tips and toothed margins extending three-quarters of the way down the leaflet leaving a smooth leaf base. They are thin and have a smooth texture. Flowers are small, creamy white, five-petaled and measure three-eighths inch wide. They bloom in bunched, flat-topped clusters and have an unpleasant scent. Fruits are small, soft berries measuring three-eighths inch in diameter. They are green when young, turning shades of yellow-orange and red when ripe. Flavor quality is very poor being dry, mealy and extremely bitter. Seeds are small, soft and numerous.

Habitat: clearings, parks, roadsides.

Medicinal parts: inner bark, flowers, berries.

Harvest: spring, inner bark; late spring–early summer, flowers; late summer–fall, berries.

Medicinal uses: dried inner bark tea for diarrhea, female complaints; fresh or dried flowers for constipation, kidney disorders, female complaints, to promote urine flow; fresh berry tea for constipation, kidney or gall bladder disorders, indigestion, sore throat, diarrhea, female complaints, to promote urine flow; fresh berry ointment for hemorrhoids.

Warning! Seeds are suspected to contain amounts of hydrogen cyanide, which causes vomiting and possibly death if eaten in quantity; their use is not recommended.

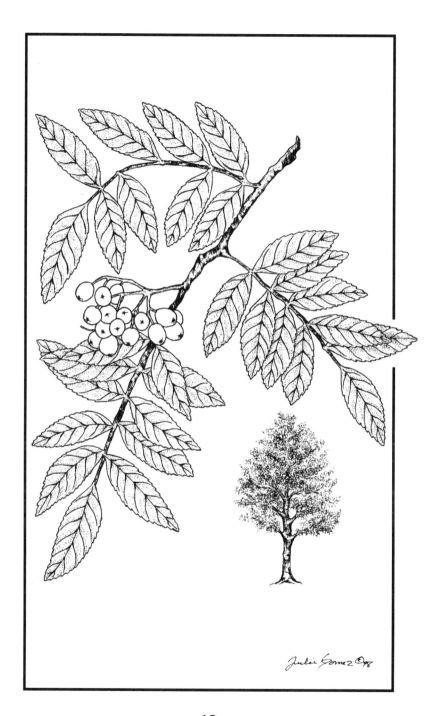

Julie Gomez ©98

15

Flowering Dogwood *Cornus florida*

Flowers: pinkish white; bloom April–June.
Fruit: red; August–November.
Life cycle: deciduous tree.
Size: fifteen to thirty feet tall.

A lovely slow-growing tree often planted as an ornamental, it has been successfully introduced into the wild through planting. Its bark is dark brown and smooth in young trees, while older trees develop a reddish gray-brown bark that is rough with scalelike patterns. Leaves grow opposite and measure three to six inches long. They are dark green above, pale green below and reveal prominent veins. Their shape is broadly ovate with wavy margins and a blunt tip. Short-stemmed, they form bush clusters on dark twigs that reveal numerous leaf scars. They are somewhat thick and have a smooth texture. Flowers bloom in showy clusters. They are pinkish white having four, notched, petal-like bracts and measure three to four inches wide. Fruits develop in bunched clusters. They are scarlet red, oblong-shaped, have blackened tips and measure one-half inch in diameter. Flavor is of very poor quality being dry and bitter. Seeds are a two-seeded nutlet.

Habitat: dry woods, parks, gardens, roadsides.

Medicinal parts: root bark, inner bark, flowers, fruit.

Harvest: spring, root bark, inner bark, flowers; late summer–fall, fruit.

Medicinal uses: dried root bark tea, tincture or powder for indigestion, diarrhea, fever, pneumonia; inner bark poultice for external ulcers; fresh or dried flower tea for indigestion, diarrhea, fever, pneumonia; fresh fruit tea or tincture for indigestion, to aid digestion.

Warning! There is some discrepancy as to whether or not fruit is poisonous. Sources indicate it may be poisonous to some degree; thus, it should not be eaten in quantity.

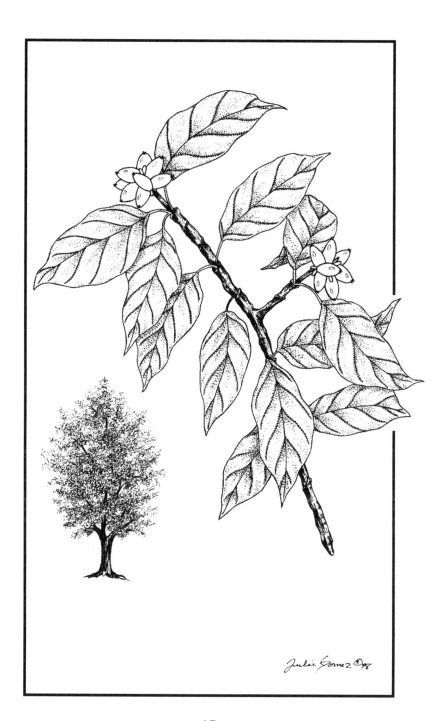

Julie Gomez ©98

Nootka Rose *Rosa nutkana*

Flowers: pink; bloom May–July.
Fruit: orange to red; July–November.
Life cycle: deciduous shrub.
Size: three to six feet tall.

This sweet-scented shrub is a favorite. The bark is deep, reddish brown and often reveals pairs of thorns located at the base of the leaves. (Some plants may have less thorns than others or none at all.) Leaves are compound and alternate. Leaflets are ovate, number from five to seven per compound and measure one to two and three-quarter inches long. They are bright green above, pale green below. They have rounded tips, shallow-toothed margins and a thin, smooth texture. Flowers are large, pink, five-petaled and measure one to three inches wide. They bloom solitary at ends of branches and are sweet scented. Fruits (also called hips or rose berries) are bright orange or red, somewhat pear-shaped and reveal five long sepals. They measure one-quarter to one and one-half inches long. Their flavor is bitterly sweet, but tolerable. Seeds are small, soft and numerous, and are coated with fuzzy hairs.

Habitat: forests, deciduous woods, clearings, hillsides, thickets, lake edges, stream and river banks, roadsides.

Medicinal parts: inner bark, leaves, petals, fruits, seeds.

Harvest: spring–summer, inner bark; spring–summer, shoots, leaves, flower petals; fall–winter, fruits, seeds.

Medicinal uses: fresh inner bark for eyewash; leaf poultice for sore eyes, abscesses, insect bites and stings; fresh flower petal tea for diarrhea; fresh or dried fruit tea for colds, stomachaches, diarrhea, scurvy; seed tea (with hairs removed!) for healthy membrane tissue, healthy red blood cells.

Warning! Always remove fuzzy seed hairs before use; they can severly irritate the mouth, throat and digestive tract!

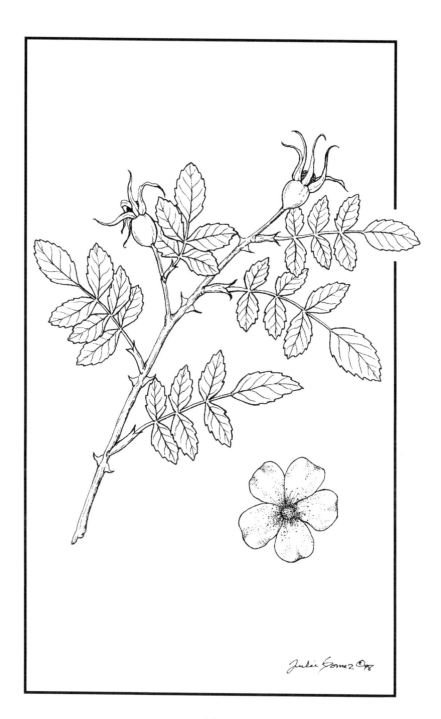

Serviceberry *Amelanchier alnifolia*

Flowers: white; bloom April–June.
Fruit: blue-black; July–August.
Life cycle: deciduous shrub or tree.
Size: sixteen feet tall.

A spreading, bushy shrub or tree that produces applelike blossoms and alderlike leaves. Its bark is reddish brown to grayish brown with a reddish hue that may or may not be smooth. Leaves alternate and measure two inches long. Above, they are dark green and pale green below. They are long-stemmed, ovate-shaped with rounded tips and reveal toothed margins that extend three-quarters of the way down the leaf (leaving a smooth margin that extends down to the leaf base). They are thin and have a smooth texture. Flowers are large and showy, and bloom in clusters that are pink at first, turning blue-black when ripe. They are round and coated with a white, waxy bloom. They measure one-quarter to one-half inch in diameter. Flavor quality is good; they are sweet and juicy, and have a slight applelike flavor. Seeds are hard and occur in pairs in the center of the fruit's core.

Habitat: forest openings, thickets, meadows, hillsides, prairies, swampy places, lake and stream edges, roadsides.

Medicinal parts: inner bark, outer bark, fruit.

Harvest: spring, inner bark, outer bark; summer, leaves; summer, fruit.

Medicinal uses: fresh inner bark wash for treating sore eyes, earache; fresh inner bark tea for diarrhea, female complaints; fresh outer bark tea for expelling worms; fresh fruit for constipation, stomach complaints.

Notice! The fruit is sometimes confused with Indian plum (*Oemleria cerasiformis*) which has a single stone and bitter taste, but is nonpoisonous.

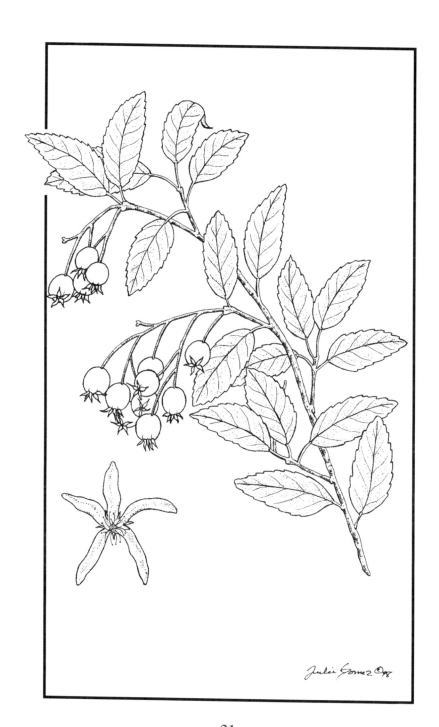

Smooth Sumach *Rhus glabra*

Flowers: greenish white; bloom June–August.
Fruit: red; September–October.
Life cycle: deciduous shrub or tree.
Size: six to fifteen feet tall.

A hardy plant, it often forms dense thickets. Its bark is smooth and pale gray (often with a reddish hue) and exudes a milky liquid, when broken, that dries into a gumlike substance. Leaves are compound and alternate on smooth, reddish, drooping limbs that seep liquid if torn. Leaflets are lance-shaped, number from eleven to thirteen (per compound) and measure two to two and one-half inches long. They have pointed tips and sharp-toothed margins. Above, they are shiny green, whitish gray below. They are thin with a smooth texture. Flowers are minute, greenish white (occasionally greenish red) and bloom in big, dense, cone-shaped clusters. Fruits are round, bright red, hairy and develop in cone-shaped clusters. Fruit diameter is one-eighth to one-quarter inch. Flavor quality is good, somewhat tart and lemony. The seed is a smooth stone.

Habitat: fields, thickets, stream banks, old farms.

Medicinal parts: root, root bark, inner trunk bark, leaves, fruit.

Harvest: spring, root, root bark, inner trunk bark; spring–summer, shoots, leaves; fall, fruit.

Medicinal uses: root tea to promote urine flow, induce vomiting; dried root bark tea for fever, sore throat, diarrhea, antiseptic, tonic; powdered root bark poultice is antiseptic; dried inner trunk bark tea for mouth and throat ulcers, fever, diarrhea, tuberculosis, antiseptic, tonic, female complaints; leaf tea for mouth disease, asthma, diarrhea; fruit tea to promote urine flow.

Warning! Sources indicate roots and shoots may cause toxic poisoning; their uses aren't recommended. Do not confuse with poison sumach (a deadly species!), which has leaves with toothless margins and smooth, white fruit.

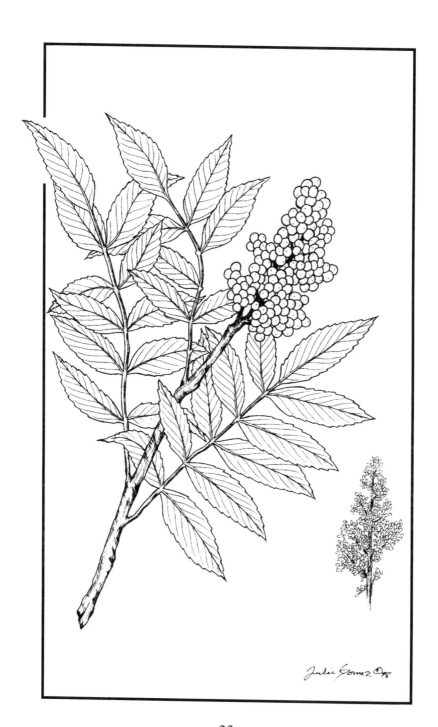

Julie Gomez '98

23

Chokecherry *Prunus virginiana*

Flowers: white; bloom April–July.
Fruit: reddish purple; July–October.
Life cycle: deciduous shrub or tree.
Size: six to twenty feet tall.

A common plant, it typically produces bushy foliage. Bark has an unpleasant odor and is grayish brown with shallow crevices that turn rough and scaly with age. Leaves alternate, measuring two to four inches long. They are shiny dark green above and below. They are ovate-shaped with pointed tips, have sharp-toothed margins and are supported by long, reddish leaf stalks. They are thin with a smooth texture. Flowers are white, five-petaled and measure a half inch wide. They hang in long, drooping, clusters measuring three to six inches long. Fruit are small, round, reddish purple and cherrylike. They appear in grapelike clusters measuring one-quarter to one-half inch in diameter. Flavor quality is poor to fair; some are mild and sweetly tart, while others are very bitter. The seed is a small, oval stone.

Habitat: woodland margins, fields, thickets, stream banks, roadsides.

Medicinal parts: root, inner bark, fruit.

Harvest: fall, root, inner bark; late summer–fall, fruit.

Medicinal uses: dried root tea as appetite stimulant, sleep inducer, blood tonic; dried inner bark tea for headaches, fever, congestion, sore throat, inflamed gums, diarrhea, asthma, ulcers, inducing sleep, disinfectant tonic; dried bark tea gargle for sore throats; fresh inner bark poultice for burns, sores, abrasions, dried or powdered fruit for diarrhea, bloody bowels, appetite stimulant.

Warning! Leaves contain cyanide and are extremely poisonous and should never be used! Sources indicate that the bark and seeds may also contain traces of cyanide. Excessive or prolonged use could lead to fatal poisoning; their use is not recommended.

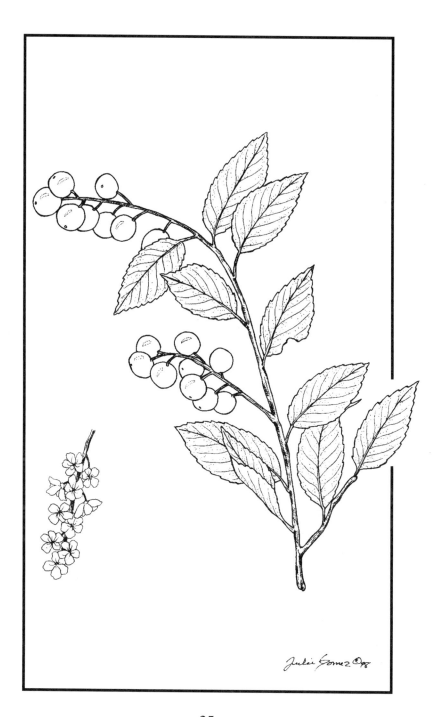

Trailing Blackberry *Rubus ursinus*

Flowers: white or pink; bloom June–July.
Fruit: black; July–August.
Life cycle: deciduous shrub.
Size: one-half to two feet tall.

This low, thorny shrub is the Pacific Nothwest's only native blackberry. Cane bark is greenish brown with a reddish hue and covered with sharp, recurved thorns. Canes develop rapidly, twisting and trailing across the ground, intertwining with one another causing the plant to look like a shrub. Leaves are compound and alternate. Leaflets occur in threes and measure two and one-half to four and one-half inches long. The lower pair are ovate with pointed tips and deeply toothed margins, while the upper (terminal leaflet) has deeply toothed, lobed margins. They are dark green above, pale green below with a thin, fuzzy texture. Flowers are typically white but may be pink. They are five-petaled and bloom in loose, flat-topped clusters from the leaf axils and measure one-half inch wide. Fruits are black, hairy, cone-shaped measuring one-quarter to three-quarters inch long. Flavor quality is excellent, being sweet and juicy. Seeds are hard, small and numerous.

Habitat: open woods, canyons, fields, thicket, disturbed areas, recovering logged areas, coastal areas, roadsides.

Medicinal parts: root, root bark, leaves, fruit.

Harvest: fall, root, root bark; spring–summer, shoots; summer–fall, leaves; summer, fruit.

Medicinal uses: dried root tea for sore throats, stomachaches, diarrhea, back pain; dried root bark tea for diarrhea, tonic; dried leaf tea for fever, mouth sores, diarrhea, to promote urine flow; dried leaf tea wash for hemorrhoids; fresh fruit for fever, stomachaches, diarrhea, vomiting, to aid digestion.

Warning! Use only fresh or thoroughly dried leaves since wilted leaves contain toxins that can be harmful if ingested. Wear gloves when harvesting to avoid cuts and scratches.

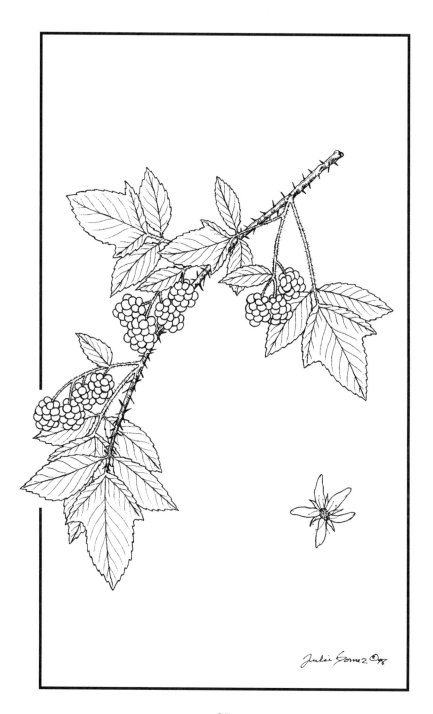

Thimbleberry *Rubus parviflorus*

Flowers: white; bloom May–July.
Fruit: red; July–September.
Life cycle: deciduous shrub.
Size: four to six feet tall.

A big-leafed shrub that is covered with fine, fuzzy hairs. The cane bark is woody, has a reddish hue and is somewhat rough and scaly. Leaves are maplelike and alternate. They are as long as they are wide and measure two to six inches. They are five-lobed, have sharp-toothed margins and are supported by long stems that give them an airy appeal. Above and below, leaves are bright green. Thin-skinned, they have a soft velvety texture. Flowers are large, white and conspicuous, and measure one and one-half to two inches wide. They are five-petaled, long-stemmed and bloom in loose, spreading clusters. Fruits are soft, dark red, raspberrylike and measure three-quarters inch in diameter. Although the fruit tends to ripen unevenly, its flavor is of good quality being sweet and juicy. Seeds are small, hard and numerous.

Habitat: open forests, clearings, thickets, stream and river banks, roadsides.

Medicinal parts: root, can bark, leaves, leaf stems, fruit.

Harvest: fall, root; summer–fall, cane bark; spring–summer, shoots, flowers leaves, leaf stems; summer–fall, fruit.

Medicinal uses: dried root tea for diarrhea; dried cane bark for diarrhea; dried leaf tea for diarrhea, anemia, to induce sleep, promote urine flow; dried, powdered leaf poultice for burns; dried, powdered leaf stem poultice for minor skin abrasions; fresh fruit and juice for diarrhea, fevers, stomachaches, scurvy.

Warning! Use only fresh or thoroughly dried leaves, since wilted leaves can release toxic compounds that can be harmful if ingested.

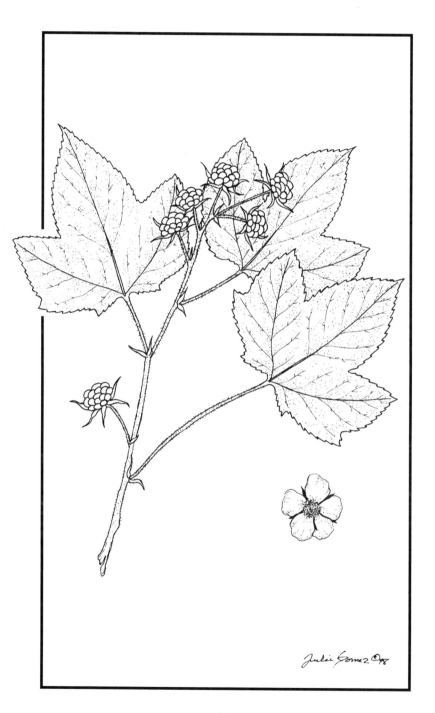

Red Huckleberry *Vaccinium parvifolium*

Flowers: greenish yellow to pink; bloom March–May.
Fruit: red; June–August.
Life cycle: deciduous-evergreen shrub.
Size: three to eight feet tall.

While hiking a forest path, shadowed by towering
conifers, I would have missed seeing this plant entirely
had it not been for its bright red berries that glowed
through the ferns. The entire plant is bright green and
slightly hairy when young, turning smooth with age.
Leaves alternate, they are ovate-shaped and generally
have smooth margins, while young leaves are occasionally
toothed. They measure one-half to three-quarters inch
long and are thin and have a paperlike texture. Flowers
are small, yellowish green blossoms that reveal pale
shades of pink and measure one-eighth inch long. They
are bell-shaped and bloom single in the leaf axils. Fruits
are small red berries that have a translucent glow and
measure one-quarter inch in diameter. Flavor quality is
good, being mildly sweet, only slightly tart and very juicy.
Dried berries have a sweeter flavor. Seeds are small, soft
and numerous.

Habitat: coniferous forest openings, forest edges, nurse
logs.

Medicinal parts: root bark, leaves, berries and juice.

Harvest: fall, root bark; summer, leaves, berries, juice.

Medicinal uses: dried root bark tea for colds, sore
throats, inflamed gums, intestinal gas, antiseptic; dried
leaf tea for sore throats, inflamed gums, diarrhea, kidney
inflammation, lower blood sugar, blood purifier, to promote urine flow; dried berry tea for diarrhea; berry juice
as an appetite stimulant.

Warning! Excessive use of fresh berries may cause ill side
effects in some.

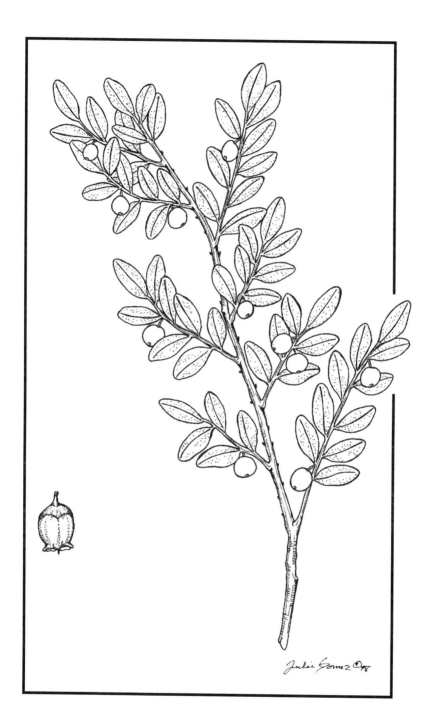

Julie Gomez ©98

31

Dwarf Blueberry *Vaccinium caespitosum*

Flowers: whitish pink; bloom June–July.
Fruit: blue; July–September.
Life cycle: deciduous shrub.
Size: one foot tall.

A small, attractive ground cover, it is easily overlooked due to its habit of growing in out of the way places. Once located, remember the place so you will be able to return to it again, since this is one plant worth coming back for. Its bark is yellowish green often with a reddish hue, and may or may not be hairy. Leaves alternate, they are short-stemmed and measure one-half inch long. Above and below they are bright green and glossy, and heavily veined below. They are lance-shaped with blunt tips, have a wedge-shaped base, and shallow-toothed margins. They are thick with a leathery texture. Flowers are small, whitish pink and measure one-eighth inch long. They are bell-shaped and look as though they bloom in clusters when really they bloom single from the leaf axils. Fruits are round, dark, blue-colored berries that are coated by a white powdery bloom and measure one-eighth inch to one-quarter inch in diameter. Flavor quality is very good being sweet and juicy. Seeds are small, soft and numerous.

Habitat: moist-wet alpine tundra, subalpine meadows, rocky slopes, bogs.

Medicinal parts: leaves, berries.

Harvest: summer, leaves; summer–fall, berries.

Medicinal uses: fresh leaf tea for diarrhea, intestinal gas, lower blood sugar, antiseptic; dried berry tea for diarrhea.

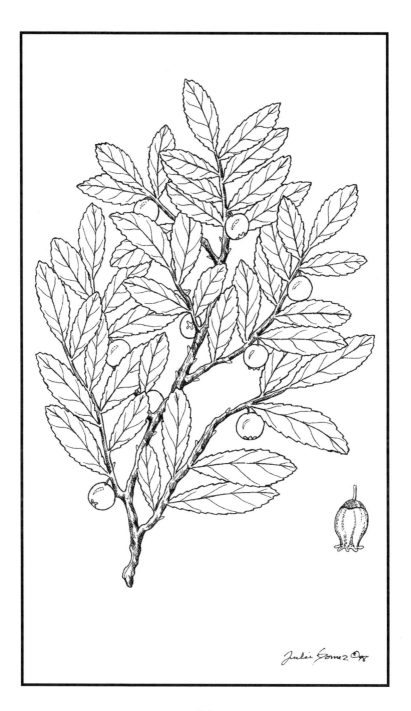

Julie Gomez ©98

Bog Blueberry *Vaccinium uliginosum*

Flowers: pinkish white; bloom June–July.
Fruit: blue-black; July–September.
Life cycle: deciduous shrub.
Size: two feet tall.

This small shrub generally has spreading branches that often form low, dense, spreading mats. Because of its small size it may be difficult to locate, but is well worth the effort. The bark is hairy and yellowish green in young plants, later turning reddish gray and becoming somewhat shredded. Leaves alternate, they are short and measure one-quarter to one and one-quarter inches long. Above, they are dark green; below they are pale green with prominent veins. They are ovate-shaped with rounded tips, have a slender base and reveal smooth margins. They are thick skinned and have a leathery texture. Flowers are small, pinkish white and measure one-eighth inch long. They are round to urn-shaped, number from two to four and bloom in loose, drooping clusters in the leaf axils. Fruits are round, blue-black berries that are coated with a white, waxy bloom and measure one-quarter to three-quarters inch in diameter. Flavor quality is very good, being sweet and juicy. Seeds are small, soft and numerous.

Habitat: moist-rocky mountain slopes, alpine tundra, subalpine meadow, bogs.

Medicinal parts: leaves, berries.

Harvest: summer, leaves; summer–fall, berries.

Medicinal uses: fresh leaf tea for diarrhea, intestinal gas, lower blood sugar, antiseptic; dried berry tea for diarrhea.

Warning! Excessive or prolonged use of the berries may cause headaches in some.

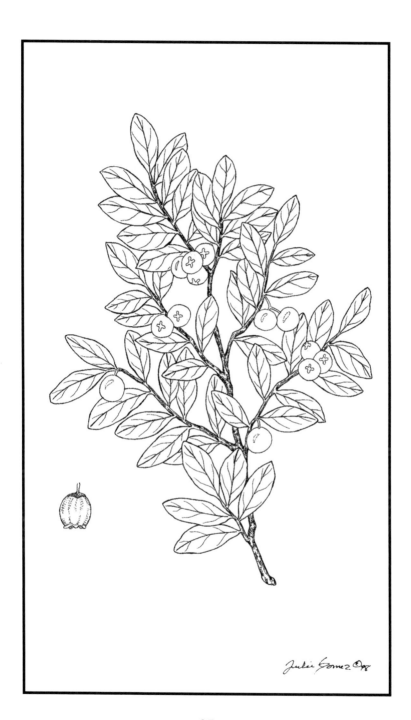

Oval-leaved Blueberry *Vaccinium ovalifolium*

Flowers: whitish pink; bloom June.
Fruit: blue-black; July–August.
Life cycle: deciduous shrub.
Size: five feet tall.

You may not have to hike as far to sample the berries of this plant since it tends to grow at lower elevations that are generally more accessible. The bark of young plants is reddish brown with a yellowish hue, while the bark of older plants is typically rough and grayish brown. Leaves alternate and measure one to two inches long. Above, they are dark green, and pale green below. Broadly ovate, they have smooth margins (although wavy margins are not uncommon). They are thick skinned and have a smooth, leathery texture. Flowers are small, whitish pink and measure three-sixteenths inch long. They are attractive, globular-shaped bells that bloom single in the leaf axils (usually before the leaves develop). Fruits are blue-black berries that measure three-eights inch in diameter and are coated with a grayish, powdery bloom. Flavor quality is very good since they are sweet and juicy. Seeds are small, soft and numerous.

Habitat: coniferous forests, open woods, thickets, bogs.

Medicinal parts: berries.

Harvest: summer, berries.

Medicinal uses: fresh or dried berry tea for diarrhea, intestinal gas, lowers blood sugar, antiseptic.

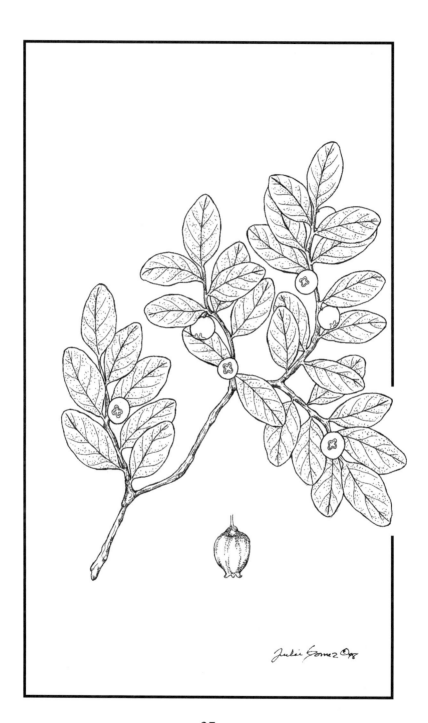

Blue Elderberry *Sambucus caerulea*

Flowers: yellowish white; bloom June–September.
Fruit: blue-black; August–September.
Life cycle: deciduous shrub or small tree.
Size: five to twenty feet tall.

A common shrub or small tree that can be easily recognized by its bright, showy flowers that are followed by drooping clusters of dark blue berries. Its bark is reddish brown highlighted with shades of green. Leaves grow opposite on spreading limbs and measure five to eight inches long. Leaflets are long-stemmed and lance-shaped with pointed tips and have fine-toothed margins. They are dark green above, slightly paler below, and have a smooth texture. They number from five to nine (per compound) and measure two to six inches long. Flowers are minute and yellowish white. They bloom in spreading, flat-topped clusters that can measure six to eight inches wide. Fruits are small, round, blue-black berries that are coated by a powdery bloom that gives them a pale blue coloring. They measure one-quarter inch in diameter and occur in dense, drooping clusters. Flavor quality is good and somewhat reminiscent of grape. Seeds are small, hard and occur in threes.

Habitat: mountainous areas, thickets, stream banks, forest openings, gullies, roadsides.

Medicinal parts: root, inner bark, flowers and stalks, berries.

Harvest: spring, root, flowers and stalks; summer, inner bark, berries.

Medicinal uses: fresh root, inner bark and flower tea for fevers, bowel spasms, laxative; inner bark ointment for burns, rashes; dried flower stalks for insect repellent; dried berry tea for diarrhea.

Warning! Berries eaten in quantity may cause ill side effects in some.

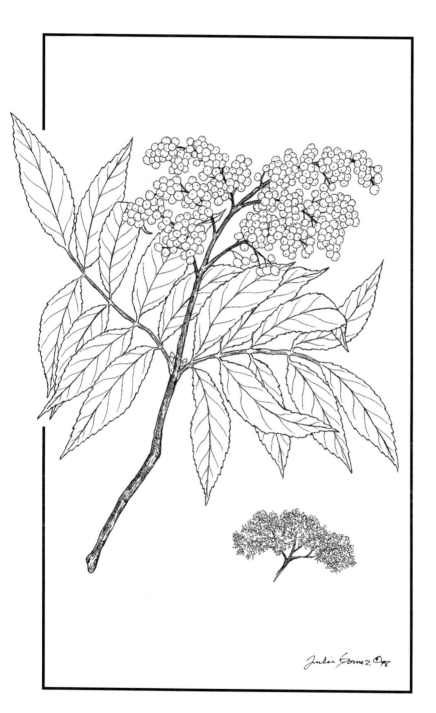

Julie Gomez ©98

39

Squashberry *Viburnum edule*

Flowers: white; bloom May–August.
Fruit: orange to red; August–October.
Life cycle: deciduous shrub.
Size: two to five feet tall.

This small shrub produces spreading limbs and has a strong, sour scent. Its bark is smooth and reddish brown in young plants, turning reddish gray with age. Leaves grow opposite and are as long as they are wide, measuring two to four inches. Above and below they are pale green and may or may not be hairy. They are three-lobed with a heart-shaped base, irregular, sharp-toothed margins and have a thin, soft, velvety texture. Flowers are minute and bright white. Short-stemmed, they bloom in loose, semi-rounded clusters that measure one-quarter to seven-sixteenths inch in diameter. They number from two to five and hang in drooping clusters. Flavor quality is poor to fair as they are quite juicy, but rather acidic and tart. The seed is a large, flattened stone.

Habitat: forests, forest edges, rocky slopes, thickets, stream banks.

Medicinal parts: bark, fruit.

Harvest: spring, bark; spring–summer, flowers; late summer–fall, fruit.

Medicinal uses: fresh bark chewed for chest colds; dried, powdered bark tea for stomachaches, female complaints; bark tea as an eyewash; fresh or dried fruit for muscular cramps, spasms, scurvy.

Warning! Raw fruit, if eaten excessively, can cause nausea.

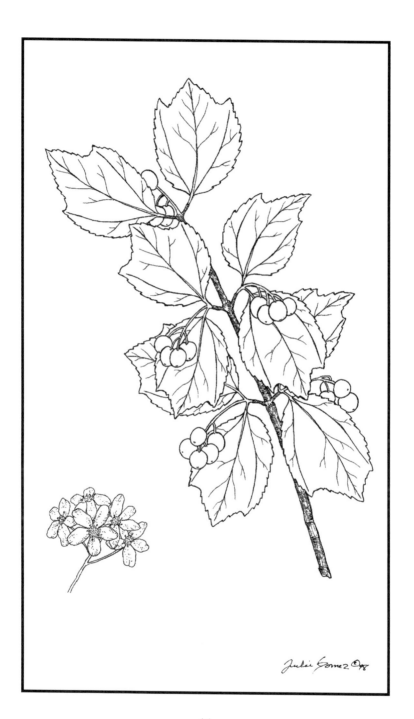

Guelder Rose *Viburnum opulus*

Flowers: white; bloom April–June.
Fruit: red; July–November.
Life cycle: deciduous shrub.
Size: five to twelve feet tall.

This tall, attractive shrub (often an ornamental) has naturalized successfully, often being mistaken for the highbush cranberry (*Viburnum trilobum*). The bark of young plants is reddish brown, turning grayish brown with age. Leaves grow opposite and measure two and one-half to four and one-half inches long. They are dark green and slightly shiny above, pale green and hairy below. Somewhat maplelike, they have three to five pointed, toothed lobes. The leaf base is smooth, broad and square-shaped. Their texture is thin, soft and velvety. Flowers are white and bloom in tight, semirounded clusters measuring four inches wide. Inner flowers are tiny replicas of the outer five-petaled flowers measuring three-quarters inch wide. Fruits appear in showy, drooping cluster. They are round to egg-shaped, bright red and translucent, measuring three-eighths inch in diameter. Their flavor quality is poor—very bitter with a disagreeable odor. The seed is a single, large stone.

Habitat: moist woods, thickets, stream bank, gardens.

Medicinal parts: bark, leaves, fruit.

Harvest: spring–fall, bark; summer, leaves; summer–winter, fruit.

Medicinal uses: dried bark chewed for muscle cramps, spasms, diarrhea, sedative, female complaints; dried leaf tea for scurvy, to induce vomiting, laxative; fresh or dried, powdered fruit tea for colds, coughs, lowering blood pressure, scurvy, stomach ulcers, laxative, urinary infection, to induce vomiting.

Warning! Conflicting sources indicate fruit may or may not be poisonous. Unripe fruit may cause nausea. Avoid eating the ripened fruit in large quantities; it may cause vomiting, stomach cramps and diarrhea.

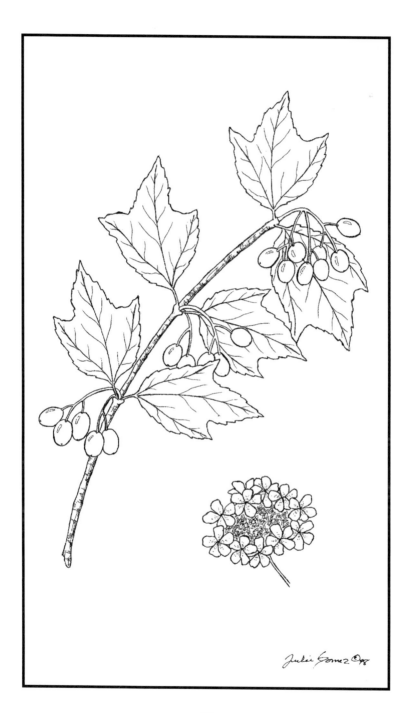

Julie Gomez ©98

Buffalo Berry *Sherpherdia canadensis*

Flowers: yellow-green; bloom April–June.
Fruit: orange-red; July–September.
Life cycle: deciduous shrub.
Size: three to nine feet tall.

This is typically a low, spreading shrub that is easy to recognize due to its unique foliage and fruit. Its bark is grayish brown and reveals reddish brown scales. Leaves grow opposite and measure one-half to one and one-half inches long. Above, the leaves are dark green, while below they are hairy, silver-green and peppered with reddish brown scales. Short-stemmed, they are ovate-shaped with rounded tips and smooth margins. They are thin and have a slight, fuzzy texture. Flowers bloom in inconspicuous clusters from the leaf axils. They are small, yellowish green bells that measure one-sixteenth to one-eighth inch long. Fruits develop in the leaf axils and appear in bunched clusters. They are ovate-shaped, bright orange-red, translucent and have a filmy texture. They measure one-half inch in diameter. Flavor quality is poor (especially in fresh fruit). Although juicy, they are extremely bitter and rather soapy. The seed is a single stone.

Habitat: rocky-sandy soils, burnt ground, forest openings, thickets, stream banks.

Medicinal parts: fruit.

Harvest: summer, fruit.

Medicinal uses: fresh fruit tea for constipation.

Warning! Fruits contain saponin (a natural sugar common in plants that makes a frothy foam when mixed with water) that can cause stomach upset if eaten in excess or in quantity.

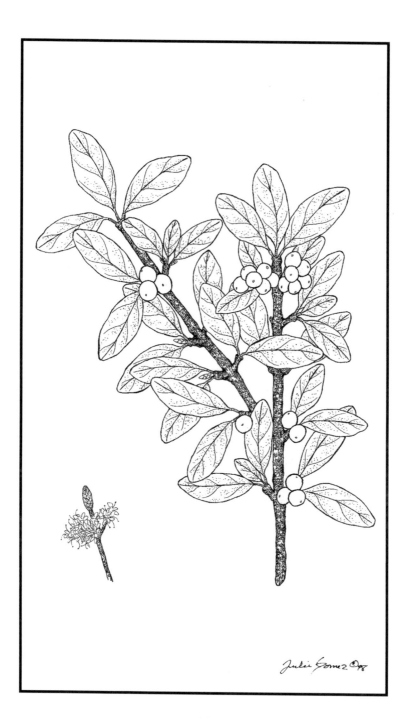

Dull Oregon Grape   *Berberis (Mahonia) nervosa*

Flowers: yellow; bloom April–June.
Fruit: blue; July–September.
Life cycle: evergreen shrub.
Size: one to two feet tall.

This attractive, upright shrub is easy to recognize due to its distinct hollylike leaves. Because it is a hardy plant, it can be easily propagated from seed or obtained from nursery stock for planting in the garden. Its bark is reddish to yellowish brown and has a very coarse texture. Leaves are compound and alternate on stiff, upright limbs measuring six to fifteen inches long. Leaflets are oblong, hollylike with sharp, spiny margins. Above, they are shiny dark green, and dull green below. They number from nine to nineteen (per compound) and measure two to three and one-half inches long. They are thick and have a smooth, leathery texture. Flowers are bright yellow, very small and bloom in dense, upright clusters measuring from three to eight inches long. Fruits are round and develop in upright clusters. They are dark blue underneath a white powder bloom and measure one-quarter inch in diameter. Flavor quality is poor to fair; they are very tart, but have a somewhat lemony flavor. Seeds are small, hard and numerous.

Habitat: dry-moist forests, forest openings, rocky slopes, roadsides, parks, gardens.

Medicinal parts: root, root bark, berries.

Harvest: spring–summer, leaves; summer, berries; fall, root, root bark.

Medicinal uses: dried root tea for coughs, acne, eczema, psoriasis, blood tonic, stomachaches, mild laxative, to aid digestion, promote urine flow; dried root bark tea for coughs, headaches, stomachaches, mild laxative, aid digestion, liver and gall bladder complaints, blood and spleen tonic; fresh or dried berry teas for fevers, gall bladder complaints, liver tonic, scurvy.

46

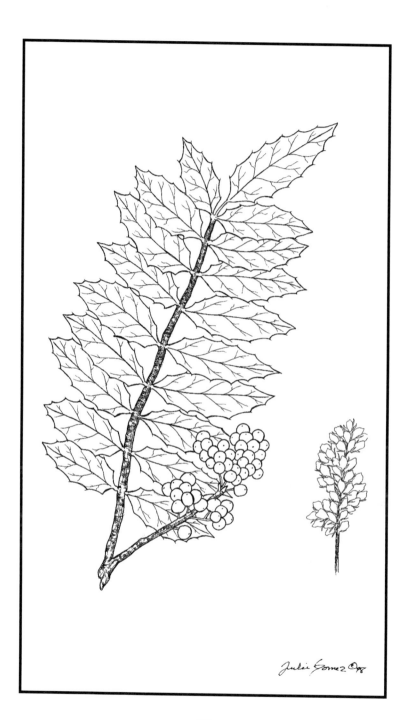

Julie Gomez ©98

Cowberry *Vaccinium vitis-idaea*

Flowers: pink to red; bloom June–July.
Fruit: red; August–October.
Life cycle: evergreen shrub.
Size: four to ten inches tall.

A low, slender-branched, evergreen shrub that has naturalized successfully and forms upright, spreading mats from creeping rhizomes. The bark is reddish brown and slightly hairy. Leaves alternate on slender limbs and measure one-quarter to three-quarters inch long. Above, they are dark green, shiny and have a furrowed midrib. Below, they are pale green and reveal dark, hairy flecks. They are ovate-shaped with inward curled margins and are short-stemmed. Thick skinned, they have a soft, leathery texture. Flowers are small and vary in color from pink to red. They are slender and bell-shaped with backward-curved lobes and measure one-quarter to five-sixteenths inch long. They bloom in short, drooping clusters. Fruits are round, bright red berries that measure one-quarter to seven-sixteenths inch in diameter. Flavor quality is poor to fair as they are somewhat juicy and rather tart at first, then become increasingly bitter. Although berries are edible as soon as they ripen, their flavor improves in the fall after the first frost. Seeds are small, soft and numerous.

Habitat: open areas, rocky soils, alpine meadows, bogs.

Medicinal parts: leaves, berries.

Harvest: early summer, leaves; summer–fall, berries.

Medicinal uses: dried leaf tea for diarrhea, kidney stones, arthritis, gout, cooling, antiseptic, diabetes to promote urine flow; fresh or dried berries for diarrhea, appetite stimulant, cooling, scurvy.

Warning! Excessive use of leaves and berries may cause nausea in some.

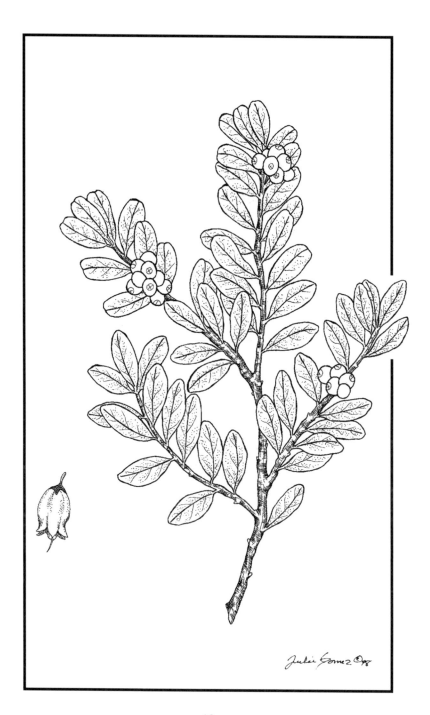

Evergreen Huckleberry *Vaccinium ovatum*

Flowers: pinkish white; bloom May–July.
Fruit: blue-black; August–December.
Life cycle: evergreen shrub.
Size: two to four feet tall.

This is a stout, bushy, sweet-scented shrub that produces attractive foliage on upright, spreading limbs. Its bark is rough and reddish brown with new growth often being hairy. Leaves alternate and measure one to two inches long. They are dark green and shiny above, and bright green below. Ovate-shaped, they have pointed tips, a prominent midrib and sharp-toothed margins. Their texture is thick, soft and leathery. Flowers are pinkish white and bell-shaped with a dark pink calyx. They are long-stemmed and bloom in drooping clusters from the leaf axils and measure one-quarter inch long. Fruits are round, shiny, blue-black berries that measure one-eighth to one-quarter inch in diameter. Flavor quality is poor to fair as they are slightly sweet and have somewhat of a musky flavor and scent. Seeds are small, soft and numerous.

Habitat: forest openings, coastal areas.

Medicinal parts: leaves, berries.

Harvest: summer, leaves; late summer–winter, berries.

Medicinal uses: fresh or dried berry tea for diarrhea, intestinal gas, lower blood sugar, antiseptic, tonic.

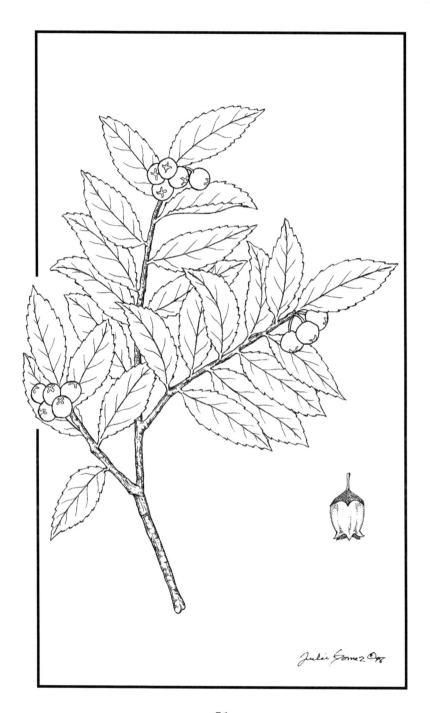

Julie Gomez ©98

Bearberry   *Arctostaphylos uva-ursi*

Flowers: pinkish white; bloom May–July.
Fruit: red; August–July.
Life cycle: evergreen shrub.
Size: three inches to one foot tall.

A low, creeping shrub that produces rooting limbs, that form dense mats across the ground. Its bark is reddish brown and coated with fine hairs. Leaves alternate on strong, flexible limbs and measure one to one and one-quarter inches long. Above, they are dark green and glossy, pale green below. They are ovate-shaped with smooth margins and have a thick skin and a smooth, waxy texture. Flowers are white to pink, urn-shaped and measure one-eighth inch long. Long-stemmed, they bloom in short drooping clusters (numbering five to twelve per cluster). Fruits are round, bright red berries that measure one-quarter to three-eighths inch in diameter. Flavor quality is very poor as they are generally bland and mealy. Flavor slightly improves upon cooking. Seeds are hard and occur in fives.

Habitat: dry rocky-sandy areas, forest openings, forest edges.

Medicinal parts: leaves, berries.

Harvest: late summer–early fall, leaves; late summer–fall, berries.

Medicinal uses: dried leaf tea for bronchitis, indigestion, diarrhea, urinary infections, kidney stones, female complaints, tonic, to induce sleep, to promote urine flow; fresh berries for kidney stones.

Warning! Excessive or prolonged use may cause nausea, constipation and possibly toxic poisoning.

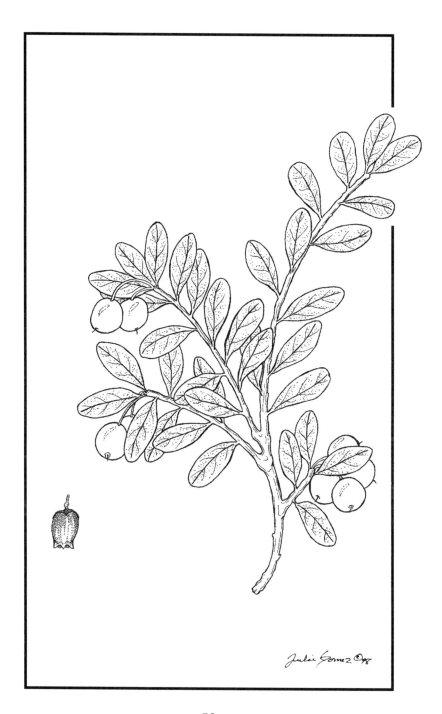

Julie Gomez '98

Ground Juniper *Juniperus communis*

Fruit: blue-black; August–October.
Life cycle: evergreen shrub.
Size: two to six feet tall.

This is typically a low, spreading shrub (rarely a tree) that grows in poor soil and can tolerate drought conditions. Its bark is reddish brown, thin, rough and peeling. Leaves are lance-shaped needles with pointed tips that occur in whorls of three and measure one-half inch long. Above, they are dark green with a distinctive white band, and pale green below. They are sharp and very stiff. Female fruits (cones) are berrylike and develop in the leaf axils. They are round, hard and green their first year, turning blue-black with a coat of white powder bloom the second year when fully ripe. They measure one-quarter to three-eighths inch in diameter. Flavor quality is good, as they are rather spicy and have a pleasant ginlike aroma and flavor. Seeds are hard and usually occur in threes.

Habitat: dry open woods, rocky slopes, dry scrub, parks, gardens.

Medicinal parts: leaves, stems, berries.

Harvest: summer–fall, leaves, stems, berries.

Medicinal uses: fresh leaf and stem tea for kidney and bladder complaints, digestive disorders, reduce swelling brought on by fluid in the cells and tissues, to promote urine flow, expel phlegm; dried berry tea for coughs, expelling intestinal parasites, digestive disorders, promotes urine flow, kidney and bladder complaints, expel intestinal gas, induce perspiration, reduce swelling brought on by fluid in the cells and tissues, antiseptic, tonic; berry ointment for arthritis, minor skin abrasions.

Warning! Excessive or prolonged use of the berries can cause digestive upsets, convulsion, kidney damage or possible kidney failure. Berry oil may cause blistering in some. Their use is not recommended.

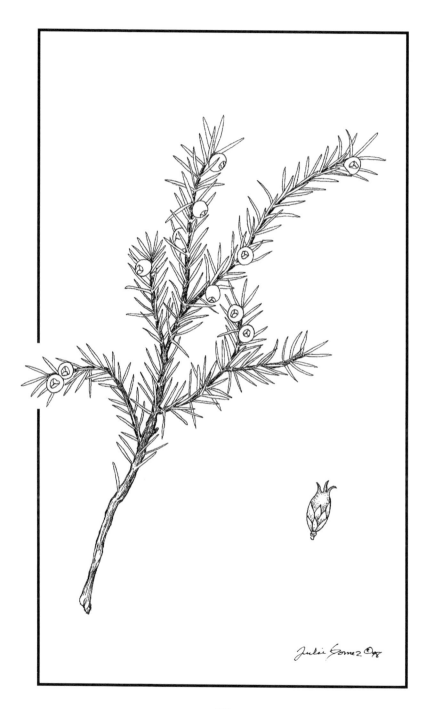

False Soloman's Seal *Smilacina racemosa*

Flowers: creamy white; bloom May–June.
Fruit: red; September–November.
Life cycle: perennial herb.
Size: one to three feet tall.

This hardy herb prefers well-drained soils and is easily transplanted or started from seed. The stalk is slender and coated with fine hairs above, while below it's smooth. It grows in a stiffened, graceful arch and has a zigzagging nature, but is nonbranching. Leaves alternate, they are short-stemmed (almost clasping the stalk) and measure three to eight inches long; above and below they are bright green. Ovate-shaped, the leaves have pointed tips, parallel veins and smooth, wavy margins. They are thin with a waxy texture. Flowers are cream-colored, short-stemmed, six-petaled and have very long stamens of one-eighth to one-quarter inch width. They bloom in showy, elongated clusters, are very fragrant and sweet scented. Fruits are round, soft, fleshy berries that are white with golden flecks at first, turning scarlet red with white or purple flecking when ripe. They measure one-eighth to one-quarter inch in diameter. Flavor quality is poor to good as fresh berries tend to be more bitter than sweet, while cooked berries tend to be sweeter. Seeds are small, hard and number three or four.

Habitat: moist coniferous and deciduous forests, clearings, stream banks.

Medicinal parts: root, leaves, berries and juice.

Harvest: spring–fall, root; spring, shoots; spring–summer, leaves; fall, berries.

Medicinal uses: root tea for constipation, kidney complaints, arthritis, female complaints; fresh root poultice for skin abrasions, sunburn; dried leaf tea for coughs, contraceptive; leaf tea wash for itching; fresh or cooked berries for constipation, scurvy; berry juice poultice for open wounds.

Warning! The root is considered poisonous and should be soaked in lye and boiled before use. Berries, if eaten in excess, can cause diarrhea. Their use is not recommended!

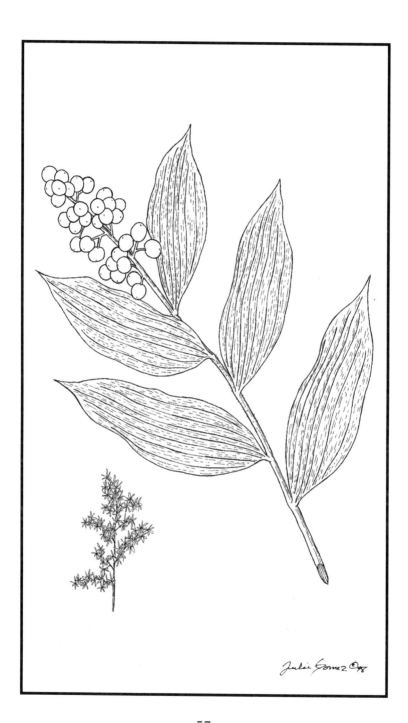

Wood Strawberry *Fragaria vesca*

Flowers: white; bloom May–June.
Fruit: red; July–August.
Life cycle: perennial herb.
Size: three to six inches tall.

Although this plant is generally abundant, its fruit is not, so I do not bother to collect it in quantity and enjoy it as a trail nibble instead. Its stalks are slender, reddish green and covered with short, stiff hairs. Leaves form a loose rosette and consist of three leaflets. They are long-stemmed and do not rise above the flowers or fruit. Leaflets are broadly ovate with pointed tips, strongly veined, have toothed margins and measure one to one and one-half inches long. They are dark green above, whitish green below and have a thin, fuzzy texture. Flowers are white with a yellow center, five-petaled and measure one-half to three-quarters inch wide. They bloom from tall, slender, hairy, upright stalks that seldom exceed six inches tall. Fruits are miniature replicas of the store-bought version. They are red, cone-shaped and reveal ten, short, green sepals. Long-stemmed they hang in drooping clusters of two or more and measure three-eighths inch in diameter. Flavor quality is excellent; they are very sweet. Seeds are soft, numerous and protrude from the fruit's fleshy, outer surface.

Habitat: rocky embankments, forest openings.

Medicinal parts: roots, leaves, fruit and juice.

Harvest: fall, root; summer, leaves, fruit and juice.

Medicinal uses: dried root tea for diarrhea, to promote urine flow; fresh or dried leaf tea for diarrhea, constipation, cooling, calming, blood tonic, scurvy, to promote urine flow; fresh leaf tea wash for sunburned skin; fresh fruit for diarrhea, constipation, tonic, to promote urine flow; fresh fruit poultice for sunburned skin; fruit juice is cooling.

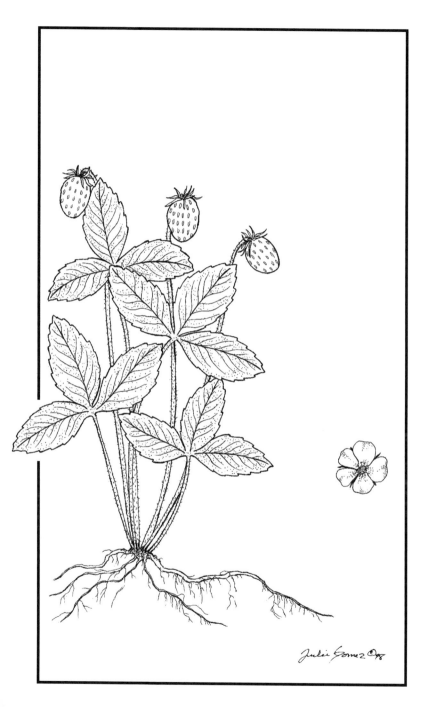

Bunchberry *Cornus canadensis*

Flowers: white; bloom April–June.
Fruit: red; June–August.
Life cycle: perennial.
Size: three to eight inches tall.

Spreading by underground rhizomes, this lovely, low trailing herb produces attractive foliage, showy flowers and bunches of conspicuous fruit. The stalk is succulent, slightly hairy, grows upright and has a woody base. Leaves occur in whorls of four to six above one or two pairs of leafy bracts and measure one and one-half to three and one-eighth inches long. Above, they are dark green with pronounced veins, while below they are whitish green. Their shape is broadly ovate with pointed tips and smooth margins. They are thin and have a smooth texture. Flowers are small, greenish white clusters that are located in the center of four large, white, petal-like bracts and measure three-quarters to one and one-half inches wide. Fruits develop in tight-bunched clusters. They are bright red, round and measure one-quarter to five-sixteenths inch in diameter. Flavor quality is poor since they are very bland and pulpy. The seed is a single stone.

Habitat: coniferous forest, forest openings, mixed woods, tree trunks, nurse logs, bogs, meadows.

Medicinal parts: roots, leaves, fruit.

Harvest: fall, root; summer, leaves, fruit.

Medicinal uses: dried root tea for infant colic; dried leaf tea for fevers, coughs, body aches, lung ailments, kidney complaints; fresh fruit as a strong laxative.

Warning! Excessive use of fruit can cause diarrhea.

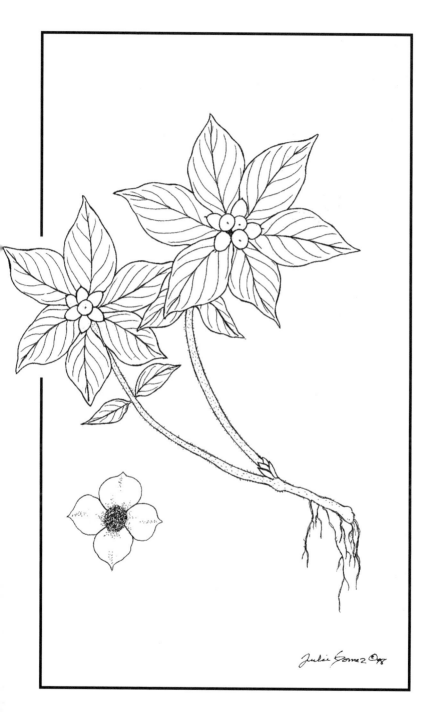

Twisted Stalk *Streptopus amplexifolius*

Flowers: greenish white; bloom May–June.
Fruit: red; August–September.
Life cycle: perennial.
Size: three to eight inches tall.

Its broad leaves often hide its delicate blossoms and handsome fruit. Its stalk grows upright and is slender, smooth and zigzagging with arched, branching stems. Leaves alternate clasping the stalk and measure two to four inches long. Above, they are dark green and pale green below. They are ovate to lance-shaped with pointed tips, have parallel veins and reveal smooth margins that are occasionally toothed. Their texture is thin and smooth. Flowers are greenish white and bell-shaped with slender, spreading petals measuring one-half inch long. They bloom single or in pairs from long, twisted stalks that join at the leaf axils. Fruits are attractive, ovate-shaped berries, typically bright red, but may also be yellow or purple and measure one-quarter to one-half inch long. Flavor quality is good; they are very juicy, somewhat sweet and have a pleasant flavor like watermelon or cucumber, depending on ripeness. Seeds are small, hard and numerous.

Habitat: coniferous forests, thickets, clearings, stream and river banks.

Medicinal parts: root, stalk, berries, juice.

Harvest: fall, root; spring–summer, shoots, stalk; late summer–fall berries, juice.

Medicinal uses: fresh root to induce labor; stalk poultice for abrasions; fresh berries for a laxative; berry ointment for skin irritation, sunburn.

Warning! Sources indicate both plant and berries are poisonous and should be avoided. Berries if eaten in quantity can cause diarrhea. (However, I have sampled both berries and plants with no effects.) Don't confuse with false hellebore (*Veratrum viride*), which can cause fatal poisoning.